About the NCCN Guidelines for Patients®

NCCN National Comprehensive Cancer Network®

Did you know that top cancer centers across the United States work together to improve cancer care? This alliance of leading cancer centers is called the National Comprehensive Cancer Network® (NCCN®).

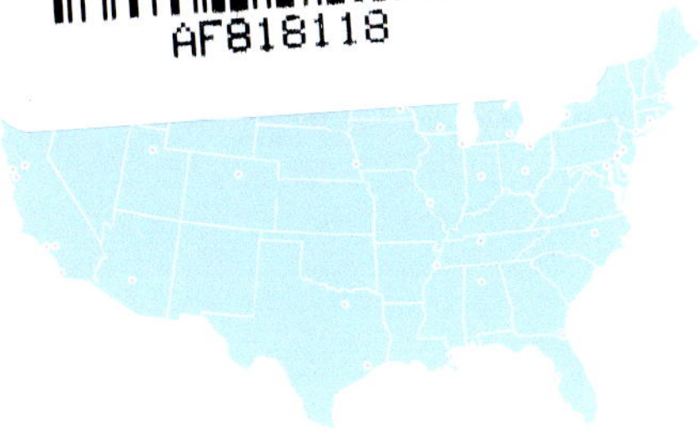

Cancer care is always changing. NCCN develops evidence-based cancer care recommendations used by health care providers worldwide. These frequently updated recommendations are the NCCN Clinical Practice Guidelines in Oncology (NCCN Guidelines®). The NCCN Guidelines for Patients plainly explain these expert recommendations for people with cancer and caregivers.

These NCCN Guidelines for Patients are based on the NCCN Clinical Practice Guidelines in Oncology (NCCN Guidelines®) for Systemic Mastocytosis, Version 1.2025 — February 21, 2025.

Learn how the NCCN Guidelines for Patients are developed
NCCN.org/patient-guidelines-process

View the NCCN Guidelines for Patients free online
NCCN.org/patientguidelines

Find an NCCN Cancer Center near you
NCCN.org/cancercenters

Connect with us

Supporters

NATIONAL COMPREHENSIVE CANCER NETWORK®
NCCN FOUNDATION
Guiding Treatment. Changing Lives.

NCCN Guidelines for Patients are supported by funding from the NCCN Foundation®

NCCN Foundation gratefully acknowledges the following corporate supporter for helping to make available these NCCN Guidelines for Patients: Blueprint Medicines.

NCCN independently adapts, updates, and hosts the NCCN Guidelines for Patients. Our corporate supporters do not participate in the development of the NCCN Guidelines for Patients and are not responsible for the content and recommendations contained therein.

To make a gift or learn more, visit online or email

NCCNFoundation.org/Donate

PatientGuidelines@NCCN.org

Contents

NCCN Foundation seeks to support the millions of patients and their families affected by a cancer diagnosis by funding and distributing NCCN Guidelines for Patients. NCCN Foundation is also committed to advancing cancer treatment by funding the nation's promising doctors at the center of innovation in cancer research. For more details and the full library of patient and caregiver resources, visit NCCN.org/patients.

National Comprehensive Cancer Network (NCCN) and NCCN Foundation
3025 Chemical Road, Suite 100, Plymouth Meeting, PA 19462 USA

1
About systemic mastocytosis

Systemic mastocytosis is a rare blood cancer that occurs when too many mast cells build up in your body. This faulty buildup can cause a variety of symptoms depending on where and how it occurs. Treatment focuses on managing symptoms and triggers. This patient guideline will break down the different types of systemic mastocytosis and how they're treated.

What is systemic mastocytosis?

Systemic mastocytosis (SM) is a rare and chronic blood cancer that happens when too many mast cells build up in your skin, tissues, and organs.

Mast cells are a type of white blood cell located throughout your body. Mast cells play a major role in your immune system and are responsible for allergic reactions.

When your immune system detects bacteria, viruses, or allergens, mast cells help fight back by releasing chemical mediators. Histamine is one of the mediators. It causes your blood vessels to expand and your skin to get itchy and swollen. It can also create a buildup of mucus, which makes the airways narrow. This response aims to protect your body from foreign invaders.

Mast cell releasing histamine

Mast cells are a type of white blood cell. They release histamine (seen here) in response to an allergen, causing an allergic reaction.

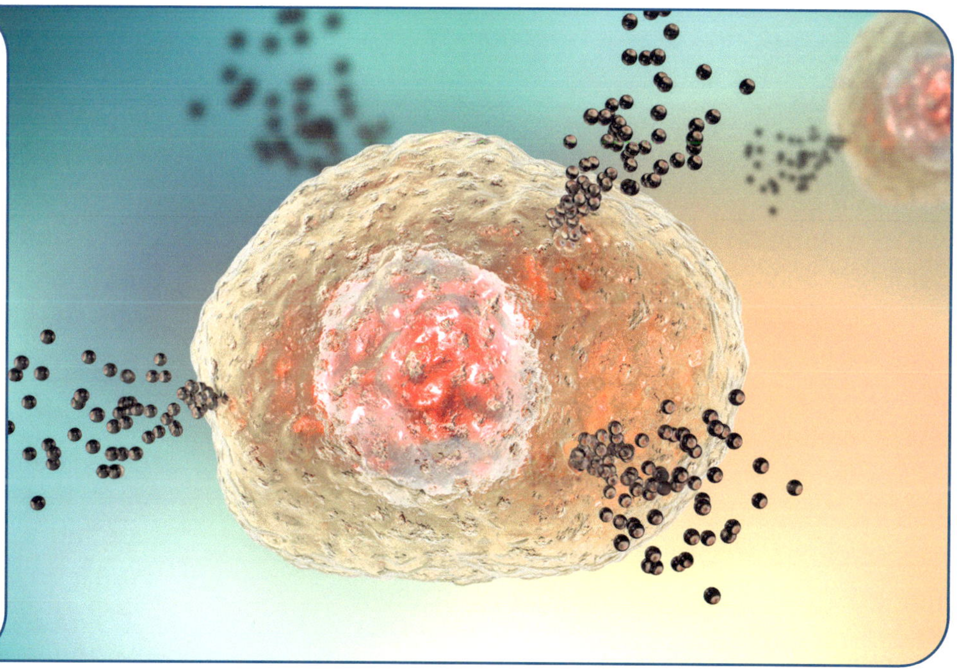

But in SM, abnormal mast cells multiply, causing inflammation and releasing histamine and other allergic mediators continuously. The oversupply of mast cells then builds up in organs like the liver, spleen, bone marrow, and gastrointestinal (GI) tract.

Much like how allergies have triggers, the same goes for SM. The difference between allergic reactions and SM is that allergic reactions are acute responses to specific allergens, and SM is a chronic disorder with abnormal mast cell buildup that can affect your organs and lead to more allergic reactions.

The symptoms of systemic mastocytosis tend to reflect where the buildup of mast cells occur. For example, mast cells that build up in the skin can cause flushing and hives, whereas mast cells that build in the GI tract can cause abdominal (belly) pain and diarrhea.

People with SM generally have an increased risk of anaphylaxis (severe, life-threatening allergic reaction) — and about half experience it. This is because they have more of the mast cells that cause the allergic reaction.

Systemic mastocytosis usually affects adults but can happen at any point in life. Another form of mastocytosis, cutaneous mastocytosis, is more common among children. This book will focus only on systemic mastocytosis.

Causes

SM is most often caused by mutations (changes) in the *KIT* gene. The *KIT* gene tells the body to make a protein that helps to control cell growth, division, survival, and movement. Mutations in this gene can cause an overproduction of mast cells. Most cases of SM are not inherited. In other words, it's an acquired or somatic mutation — happening at some point in a person's life.

Types

Once you are diagnosed with SM, it will be labeled with 1 of 5 types that include:

- **Indolent systemic mastocytosis (ISM) –** A form of systemic mastocytosis that is the most common. Most symptoms are mild. It has a low risk of progressing to more severe types of SM and does not affect survival.
    - **Bone marrow mastocytosis (BMM)** – This is a subtype of ISM where the mast cells abnormally build up in the bone marrow but not the skin or other organs. Anaphylaxis can be more severe than in ISM.
- **Smoldering systemic mastocytosis (SSM) –** While it's a milder type of SM, more mast cells build up in this type than ISM. SSM also has a higher risk of progressing to more severe disease.
- **Aggressive systemic mastocytosis (ASM) –** This type involves a higher number of mast cells building up in the body. This buildup can affect organ function (usually liver, GI tract, bone, or bone marrow).
- **Systemic mastocytosis with an associated hematologic neoplasm (SM-AHN) –** This type refers to a mast cell buildup that occurs together with another blood disorder, usually myelodysplastic syndromes, myeloproliferative disorder, or acute myeloid leukemia.

- **Mast cell leukemia (MCL)** – A very rare but aggressive cancer described as a buildup of mast cells in more than one-fifth of the body's tissues or organs.

How is systemic mastocytosis treated?

While there is no cure for SM, most people have mild to moderate symptoms that they can manage with treatments and by avoiding triggers. See *Chapter 3: Diagnosing SM.*

For information on the treatments available, see *Chapter 4: Types of treatment.*

This book also describes treatment for your specific type of systemic mastocytosis.

For common types of SM, which include ISS and SSM, see *Chapter 5: Treatment for common types of SM.*

For advanced types of SM, which include ASM, SM-AHN, and MCL, see *Chapter 6: Treatment for advanced types of SM.*

Why you should read this book

Making decisions about cancer care can be stressful. You may need to make tough decisions under pressure about complex choices.

The NCCN Guidelines for Patients are trusted by patients and providers. They clearly explain current care recommendations made by respected experts in the field. Recommendations are based on the latest research and practices at leading cancer centers.

Cancer care is not the same for everyone. By following expert recommendations for your situation, you are more likely to improve your care and have better outcomes as a result. Use this book as your guide to find the information you need to make important decisions.

What can you do to get the best care?

Advocate for yourself. You have an important role to play in your care. In fact, you're more likely to get the care you want by asking questions and making shared decisions with your care team.

The NCCN Guidelines for Patients will help you understand cancer care. With better understanding, you'll be more prepared to discuss your care with your team and share your concerns. Many people feel more satisfied when they play an active role in their care.

You may not know what to ask your care team. That's common. Each chapter in this book ends with an important section called *Questions to ask*. These suggested questions will help you get more information on all aspects of your care.

Take the next step and keep reading to learn what is the best care for you!

2 Testing

Treatment planning starts with testing. Accurate testing is part of what is needed to diagnose and treat systemic mastocytosis. This chapter presents an overview of the tests you might receive and what to expect.

Systemic mastocytosis is diagnosed based on a series of test results related to your symptoms. See the next chapter about identifying your symptoms and triggers.

To diagnose SM, biopsies (testing tissue samples) are often done to measure mast cell mediators and their appearance in the urine, blood, bone marrow, and organs. Mast cell mediators are molecules, like proteins, that are released as part of an inflammatory response. Histamine is one type of mast cell mediator.

It's important you understand what these test results mean, so be sure to ask questions.

General health tests

Medical history

A medical history is a record of all health issues and treatments you have had in your life. It gives your health care provider an overall picture of your health and that information helps guide your treatment.

For new or follow-up appointments, be prepared to list any illness or injury and when it happened. Bring a list of old and new medicines and any over-the-counter medicines, herbals, or supplements you take. Tell your health care provider about any symptoms you have. You may also want to bring in pictures of allergic skin reactions and talk about your history with them, as well as your history of anaphylaxis and potential triggers.

Family history

Some diseases can run in families. Your provider will ask about the health history of family members who are blood relatives. This information is called a family history. Ask family members about their health issues like heart disease, cancer, and diabetes, and at what age they were diagnosed.

Physical exam

During a physical exam, a provider may:

- Check your temperature, blood pressure, pulse, and breathing rate
- Check your weight and ask if you've had unexplained weight loss
- Listen to your lungs and heart
- Look in your eyes, ears, nose, and throat
- Feel and apply pressure to parts of your body to see if organs — particularly your spleen and liver — are of normal size, are soft or hard, or cause pain when touched. Tell your provider if you feel pain.
- Feel for swollen lymph nodes in your neck, underarm, and groin. Tell your provider if you have felt any lumps or have any pain.

- Conduct a complete skin exam

For a list of possible tests, see **Guide 1.**

Blood tests

Blood tests check for signs of disease and how well organs are working. They require a sample of your blood, which is removed through a needle placed into your vein.

Guide 1 Common tests for systemic mastocytosis
Medical history and physical exam, including history of mast cell activation symptoms
Comprehensive metabolic panel with uric acid, LDH, and LFTs
Serum tryptase level
CBC with differential
Examination of blood smear
Bone marrow aspirate and biopsy with flow cytometry, immunohistochemistry, and cytogenetics
FISH test
Molecular testing using a high-sensitivity assay for *KIT* D816V
Myeloid mutation panel
CT/MRI or ultrasound of the abdomen/pelvis
DEXA scan
Skeletal survey
Organ-directed biopsy
24-hour urine studies (useful in certain circumstances)
HLA testing (useful in certain circumstances)
Assessment of symptom burden and quality of life (QOL) (useful in certain circumstances)

Comprehensive metabolic panel

A comprehensive metabolic panel (CMP) is a test that measures 14 different substances in your blood. A CMP provides important information about how well your kidneys and liver are working, among other things. If those organs are not performing right, then systemic mastocytosis could be the reason.

- **Uric acid** – A uric acid blood test is a medical test used to check the amount of a normal waste product in your blood. It is also known as a serum urate test or a uric acid level.
- **Lactate dehydrogenase (LDH)** – LDH is a type of protein in blood, known as an enzyme. It is found in most of the body's tissues. When these tissues are damaged, they release LDH into the bloodstream or other body fluids. If your LDH levels are high, it may mean certain tissues in your body have been damaged by disease or injury.
- **Liver function tests (LFTs)** – LFTs look at the health of your liver by measuring chemicals that are made or processed by the liver. Levels that are too high or low signal that the liver is not working well, or the bile ducts might be blocked.

Complete blood count with differential

A complete blood count (CBC) measures the number of red blood cells, white blood cells, and platelets in your blood. Systemic mastocytosis can show as a shortage of red blood cells (anemia) or platelets (thrombocytopenia), as well as too many white blood cells (eosinophilia).

There are several types of white blood cells. A differential counts the number of each type of white blood cell. It also checks if the counts are in balance with each other.

Serum tryptase level

This type of test can help figure out if a severe allergic reaction has occurred. This test measures the amount of tryptase in the blood.

Tips to keep in mind

- Bring someone with you to your health care provider visits, if possible.
- Write down questions and take notes during appointments. Don't be afraid to ask your care team questions.
- Get copies of blood tests, imaging results, and reports about your specific disease.
- Organize your papers. Create files for insurance forms, medical records, and test results. You can do the same on your computer, if you have one.
- Keep a list of contact information for everyone on your care team. Add it to your phone. Hang the list on your refrigerator or in a place where someone can access it in an emergency. Inform your primary care physician of changes to this list.

Tryptase is an enzyme that is found in mast cells. Mast cells release histamine and other chemicals (mediators) when they are part of a normal immune response as well as an allergic reaction.

Blood smear

A blood smear is often used as further testing if your CBC shows abnormal results. This test is used to evaluate and measure the different types of blood cells as well as the presence of mast cells. It can be used to diagnose another blood disorder that's coinciding with systemic mastocytosis.

Biopsies

A biopsy is the removal of a sample of tissue or group of cells for testing. It is an important part of an accurate diagnosis. Your sample should be reviewed by a pathologist who is an expert in the diagnosis of systemic mastocytosis. The pathologist will note the overall appearance and the size, shape, and type of your cells. Tests will be done on the biopsied cells, and they are listed ahead.

Bone marrow aspiration and biopsy

Your provider might order a bone marrow aspiration and biopsy to look for increased mast cells in the bone marrow. Bone marrow is like a sponge holding liquid. A bone marrow aspiration takes some of the liquid out of the sponge; a biopsy takes a piece of the sponge. For aspiration, a hollow needle will be pushed through your skin and into the bone. Liquid bone marrow will then be drawn into a syringe. For the biopsy, a needle will be used to remove a core sample of the solid part of

Bone marrow aspiration and biopsy

Here you see a hollow needle inserted through the bone to remove a sample.

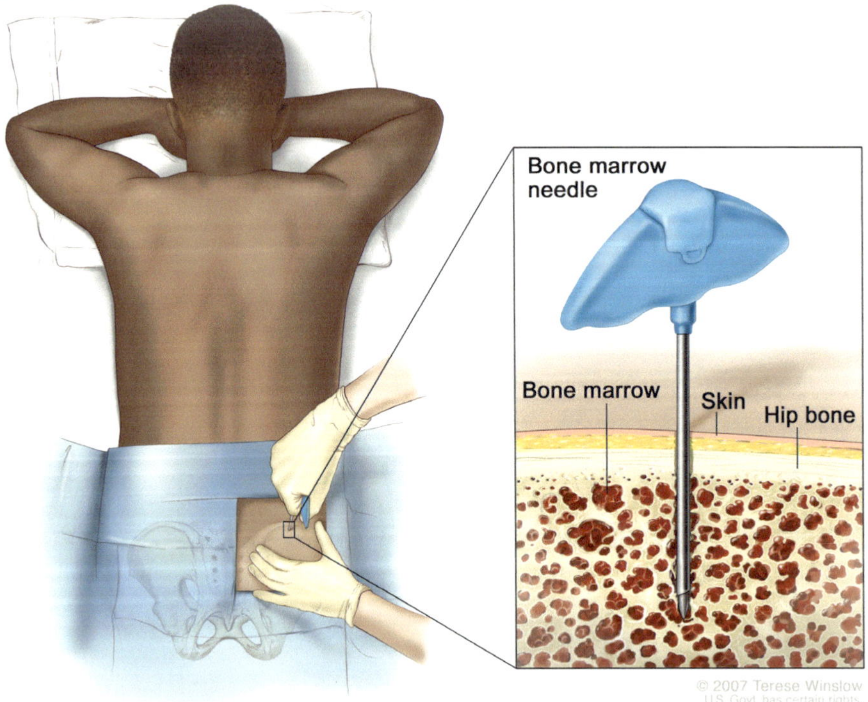

marrow. The samples will be sent to a lab for testing. You may feel pain at your hip bone for a few days. Your skin may bruise.

Ask your provider about the type of bone marrow test you might have and where the sample will be taken. Also ask if you will be given a medicine to help you relax and block any pain involved with the procedure.

Organ-directed biopsies

With systemic mastocytosis, you can expect to receive one of the following organ-directed biopsies depending on the symptoms you have.

Upper GI endoscopy

If you have abdominal symptoms (like pain, nausea, vomiting, and diarrhea), your provider might order an endoscopy. A biopsy of the upper gastrointestinal (GI) tract is often performed to confirm a diagnosis of systemic mastocytosis by looking for mast cell build up in the GI tract. This procedure uses an endoscope, a long, tube-like device with a built-in light and miniature video camera. After being given a sedative (medicine to help you relax for the procedure) and a numbing medicine for your throat, the endoscope is guided down the throat. It then goes into the esophagus, stomach, and upper parts of the small intestine. This allows your provider to inspect the lining of these organs and to look for any signs of cancer or other abnormalities such as dilated blood vessels or ulcers that can result from the buildup of mast cells. After the procedure, your throat may feel sore, and you may feel some swelling.

"Be your own advocate. Talk to someone who has gone through the same thing as you. Ask a lot of questions, even the ones you are afraid to ask. You have to protect yourself and ensure you make the best decisions for you, and get the best care for your particular situation."

Liver biopsy

An enlarged liver may be a sign of SM — but it's also a sign of many other illnesses. To help figure out the cause, your provider might order a liver biopsy. In a liver biopsy, a needle may be inserted through the skin of the abdomen to remove a liver sample. Or a needle may be inserted through a large vein in your neck (jugular) and threaded down to a vein (inferior vena cava) near your liver.

Immunophenotyping

Immunophenotyping is a type of diagnostic test that looks for the presence or absence of specific white blood cell antigens. These antigens are proteins that can be found on the surface of or inside white blood cells. They are called biomarkers.

A complete blood test can count the number of white blood cells, but it cannot detect the subtle differences between different types of blood cancers. Immunophenotyping can detect these subtle differences.

There are 2 testing methods:

- Flow cytometry
- Immunohistochemistry

Flow cytometry

Flow cytometry is a laboratory method used to detect, identify, and count specific cells. Flow cytometry involves adding a light-sensitive dye to cells. The dyed cells are passed through a laser beam in a machine. The machine measures the number of cells, the size and shape of the cells, and other unique features of cells. Flow cytometry may be used on cells from circulating (peripheral) blood or from a bone marrow aspirate.

Biomarkers of mastocytosis found by flow cytometry include the proteins CD117, CD25, CD30, and CD2.

Immunohistochemistry

Immunohistochemistry (IHC) is a special staining process that involves adding a chemical marker to cells. The cells are then studied using a microscope to identify specific proteins. Proteins that help diagnose SM include tryptase as well as CD117, CD2, CD25, and CD30.

Cells studied with flow cytometry

Dyed cells are passed through laser beams to help measure their size and shape.

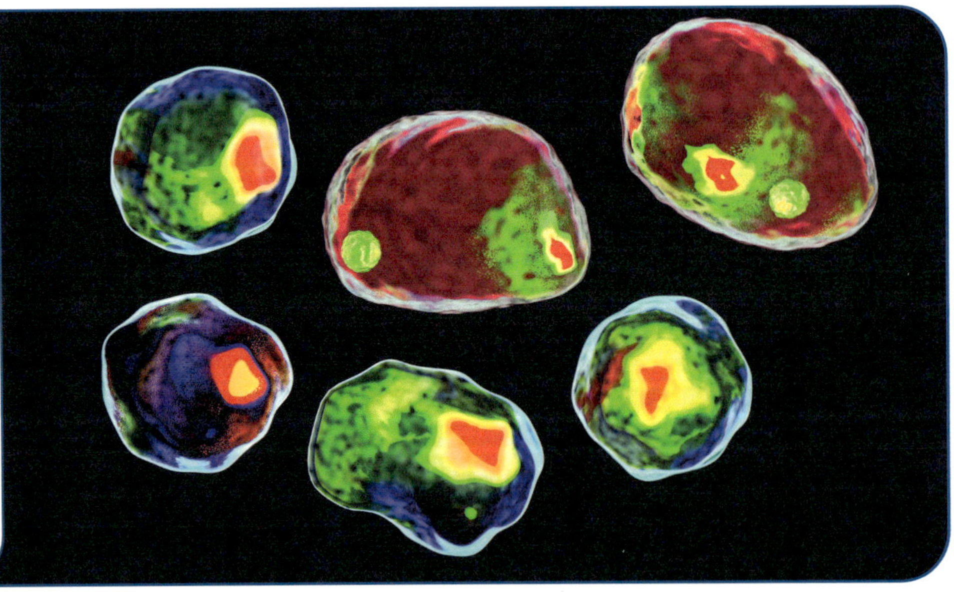

Genetic tests

Your health care provider may suggest tests for gene mutations. Genes tell cells what to become and what to do. In a process called mutation, something goes wrong in the genetic code. This can cause cells to grow and divide out of control.

Genetic testing looks for the presence or absence of certain gene mutations. They can be performed on bone marrow or a blood sample. Test results will help your treatment team learn more about your disease and make a treatment plan.

Cytogenetics

Cytogenetics is a type of genetic test that uses samples of tissue, blood, or bone marrow to look for changes in chromosomes. A chromosome is a long DNA molecule with genetic material of an organism. The test specifically looks for broken, missing, rearranged, or extra chromosomes.

Myeloid mutation panel

A myeloid mutation panel is a blood test used to identify mutated genes. This test helps to diagnose and manage diseases such as acute myeloid leukemia (AML), myelodysplastic syndrome (MDS), myeloproliferative neoplasm (MPN), and MDS/MPN. It should be noted that this panel is not sensitive enough to detect the mutation (*KIT*) that occurs with SM, so additional testing mentioned ahead is needed.

FISH test

Fluorescence in situ hybridization (FISH) is a method that involves special dyes called

Hereditary alpha-tryptasemia

Hereditary alpha-tryptasemia (HαT) refers to a genetic variant (called a polymorphism). People with HαT inherited an extra copy of the gene (TPSAB1) that makes a protein called tryptase.

Since they have extra genes making the protein, they end up with more tryptase. And too much tryptase can mean too many mast cells or systemic mastocytosis (SM).

People with SM are more likely to have HαT. But people without SM also can have it.

HαT may or may not lead to symptoms and in most cases it doesn't. But when symptoms occur they may include:

- Itchy skin, flushing, hives, and anaphylaxis
- Gastrointestinal (GI) symptoms such as bloating, abdominal pain, diarrhea and/or constipation, heartburn, and difficulty swallowing
- Connective tissue symptoms such as hypermobile joints and scoliosis
- Cardiac symptoms such as a racing or pounding heartbeat or blood pressure swings with/without fainting
- Anxiety, depression, and panic attacks

probes that attach to pieces of DNA. FISH can look for translocations (switching parts between 2 chromosomes) and inversions (switching parts within 1 chromosome) that are too small to be seen with other methods. However, it can only be used for known changes. It cannot detect all the possible changes found within your chromosomes (karyotype).

KIT gene mutations

A mutation in the *KIT* gene is the most common genetic change found in people with systemic mastocytosis. The *KIT* gene provides instructions for making a protein. It is important for the development and role of certain cell types. This includes reproductive cells (germ cells), early blood cells (hematopoietic stem cells), white blood cells (mast cells), cells in the gastrointestinal tract called interstitial cells of Cajal, and cells called melanocytes. *KIT D816V* is the gene specific to systemic mastocytosis.

Imaging

Imaging tests take pictures (images) of the inside of your body. You might need imaging to get more details about organs that might be affected and produce symptoms of systemic mastocytosis. A radiologist, an expert in interpreting test images, will write a report and send this report to your provider. Your test results will be discussed with you.

CT scan

A computed tomography (CT or CAT) scan is a computerized x-ray machine. It takes many pictures (x-rays) from different angles of the same body part. Pictures are merged to form a 3D image.

In some cases, contrast will be used. Contrast material is used to improve the pictures of the inside of the body. Contrast materials are not dyes, but substances that help enhance and improve the images of several organs and structures in the body. It is used to make the pictures clearer. Contrast might be taken by mouth (oral) or given through a vein (IV). The contrast is not permanent and will leave the body through your urine immediately after the test.

You should be instructed to drink about 8 to 10 glasses of water for 24 hours after you have the contrast. This helps to flush the contrast from your system, including the kidneys.

Tell your providers if you have had allergic reactions to contrast in the past. This is important. You might be given medicines, such as diphenhydramine (Benadryl) and prednisone (steroids) to avoid the effects of those allergies. Contrast might not be used if you have a serious allergy or if your kidneys are not working well.

MRI scan

A magnetic resonance imaging (MRI) scan uses strong magnets and radio waves to take digital pictures of the inside of the body. It does not use x-rays. Contrast might be used.

Ultrasound

An ultrasound uses high-energy sound waves to form pictures of the inside of the body. A probe will be pressed onto your abdomen. This is similar to the sonogram used for pregnancy.

Ultrasound is painless and does not use x-rays, so it can be repeated as needed. Sometimes, an ultrasound or CT is used to guide a biopsy.

DEXA scan

A DEXA scan is an imaging test that measures bone strength (density). DEXA scans are used to determine your risk for osteoporosis (bone loss) and osteopenia (weakened bones). Osteoporosis and osteopenia are common complications of mast cell build up.

Skeletal survey

A skeletal survey, also referred to as a bone survey, is a series of x-rays taken to look at all the bones in your body. This test is used to determine if bone disease is present.

Other tests

You may receive more tests such as urine testing, HLA typing, or a quality-of-life assessment. These tests will help to figure out the extent of your disease and treatment for symptoms.

Urine test

Urine tests are often used to help determine the presence of histamine in your body. The test consists of providing urine over a 24-hour period to evaluate histamine production over a longer time frame than a blood test.

HLA typing

Human leukocyte antigens (HLAs) are proteins found on the surface of most cells. They play an important role in your body's immune response.

HLAs are unique to each person. They mark your body's cells. Your body detects these markers to tell which cells are yours. Each person's set of HLAs is called the HLA type or tissue type.

HLA typing is a blood test that detects a person's HLA type. This test is done before a donor (allogeneic) blood stem cell transplant, which can be a treatment for advanced types of systemic mastocytosis.

To find a donor match, your HLA type will be compared to the donor's HLA type to see how many proteins are the same.

Quality-of-life assessment

You may be asked to complete a quality-of-life assessment. It is a questionnaire designed specifically for people with mastocytosis. It's used to identify your current physical and mental wellness, as well as your ability to function in your daily activities. It's also used to track how treatment improves or affects your quality of life.

Quality of life refers to a person's overall enjoyment of life including their sense of well-being and ability to participate in their usual activities.

What's next

This chapter gave an overview of the different types of tests that can be used to diagnose systemic mastocytosis and guide its treatment. The next chapter addresses signs and symptoms as well as triggers that need to be considered (along with test results) in your diagnosis.

Key points

- Systemic mastocytosis will be diagnosed based on a series of test results. Your diagnosis will determine your treatment plan. It is important you understand what these tests mean.
- Blood tests check for signs of disease and how well organs are working. They require a sample of your blood, which is removed through a needle placed into your vein.
- A biopsy is the removal of a sample of tissue or group of cells for testing. It is an important part of an accurate diagnosis.
- Immunophenotyping uses antibodies to detect the presence or absence of white blood cell antigens. These antigens are proteins that can be found on the surface of or inside white blood cells. They are called biomarkers.
- Genetic testing looks for the presence or absence of certain gene mutations. Test results will help your treatment team learn more about your disease and make a treatment plan.
- Imaging tests take pictures of the inside of your body.
- You may receive additional tests such as urine testing, HLA typing, or a quality-of-life assessment. These tests will help to determine the extent of your disease and treatment for symptoms.

Questions to ask

- What tests are needed? What other tests do you recommend?
- What can you do to make me comfortable during testing?
- How do I prepare for testing?
- How and where will the test be done?
- How soon will I know the results and who will explain them to me?

3
Diagnosing SM

Treatment for systemic mastocytosis depends on the diagnosis. The diagnosis depends on your disease's signs, symptoms, and triggers. After knowing your symptoms and undergoing testing, you will be diagnosed with 1 of 5 types of SM.

Signs and symptoms

Signs and symptoms of systemic mastocytosis are key to how your condition is diagnosed, managed, and treated. Symptoms of mastocytosis differ and are based on the part of the body that is affected by the buildup (accumulation) of mast cells. It's always important to let your health care provider know about any symptoms you are experiencing.

Signs and symptoms can include any or many of the following:

Skin signs and symptoms

- Flushing (skin redness and warmth)
- Macules (flat, brown or tan discolored spots less than 1 centimeter wide, which is about the width of a pencil)
- Itching
- Hives (also called urticaria; raised, itchy welts or bumps)

Gastrointestinal (GI) signs and symptoms

- Abdominal pain
- Nausea
- Vomiting
- Diarrhea

Heart signs and symptoms

- Rapid heart rate, chest pain
- Low blood pressure, which can lead to lightheadedness and fainting

Other signs and symptoms

- Wheezing, shortness of breath
- Nasal congestion and itching
- Bone pain/muscle pain
- Brain fog
- Fatigue
- Dizziness
- Frequent headaches

Signs and symptoms: What's the difference?

Signs are the effects of a health problem that other people can see (like rashes, bleeding, or swelling) and **symptoms** are those that the person experiences and others can't see (like pain, nausea, or feeling tired).

You may also experience swelling of the lymph nodes, liver and spleen, as well as anemia (low iron in your blood).

Triggers

Symptoms of mastocytosis can happen on their own (spontaneously) but they are more likely to occur if "triggered."

Common triggers can include what you eat, drink, do, or take:

- Spicy foods
- Alcohol
- Exercise
- Certain medications and vaccinations
- Surgery and other medical procedures

Triggers can also come from your environment or within your body:

- Insect stings and animal venoms
- Extreme temperatures or sudden temperature changes
- Sun/sunlight
- Natural or chemical odors
- Friction or vibrations on the skin
- Physical and emotional stress
- Infections

Complications

Effectively managing symptoms and triggers can help avoid complications from systemic mastocytosis. Complications are an unwanted result of a disease or treatment that's not well controlled. They may negatively affect outcomes. Some complications of systemic mastocytosis include:

A life-threatening anaphylactic reaction can happen as a complication of systemic mastocytosis. Your provider will want you to keep 2 injectable forms of epinephrine with you at all times.

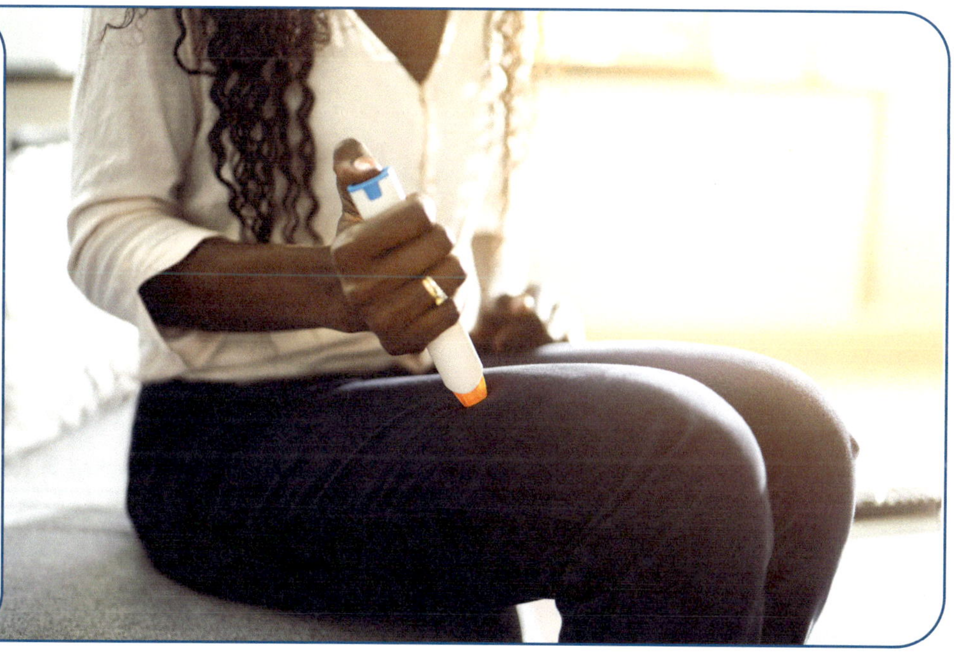

- **Anaphylactic reaction (anaphylaxis)** – rapid heartbeat, fainting, loss of consciousness, and shock. This type of severe allergic reaction may require a shot of epinephrine. An epinephrine injection is an emergency treatment for life-threatening anaphylaxis.
- **Blood disorders** – anemia (not enough red blood cells), cytopenia (low numbers of white blood cells, red blood cells and/or platelets), and poor blood clotting (not enough platelets)
- **Peptic ulcer disease** – ulcers and pain in your GI tract
- **Reduced bone density** – osteopenia and osteoporosis
- **Bone fractures** – caused by weakened bones
- **Liver, spleen, and lymph node problems** – swelling and issues with how these organs function
- **Organ failure** – swelling/enlargement and resulting damage to organs

Diagnosis

Systemic mastocytosis is often diagnosed by its signs and symptoms mentioned above, or if you experience anaphylaxis and your health care provider recommends more testing. After a physical exam, your provider may recommend a bone marrow biopsy or bone imaging, and blood and/or urine tests to measure the levels of specific chemicals or substances related to mast cells.

If tests show high levels of these substances or the presence of atypical (unusual) mast cells, you are likely to be diagnosed with SM.

You may also receive other tests to confirm or define your diagnosis. These include other types of imaging like MRI and CT scans, gastrointestinal workup, or genetic testing to confirm there is a mutation in the *KIT* gene. See *Chapter 2: Testing* for the variety of tests you could have.

Test results will identify the systemic mastocytosis as 1 of 5 types that are either common or advanced:

- Indolent SM (common)
- Smoldering SM (common)
- Aggressive SM (advanced)
- SM with associated hematologic neoplasm (advanced)
- Mast cell leukemia with or without AHN (advanced)

What's next

Once you receive your diagnosis and type of SM, you will be treated based on this information. The next chapter is an overview of the different types of treatments for SM. Keep in mind this is just an overview, and you won't receive all treatments for your type of SM. For more specific treatments, go to the chapter for your type of systemic mastocytosis (either common or advanced).

Key points

- Signs and symptoms are key to diagnosing systemic mastocytosis.
- Triggers are what can cause symptoms.
- Complications can result from symptoms that are not well controlled.
- Once tests have been completed, you will be diagnosed with 1 of 5 types of SM.

Questions to ask

- What type of mastocytosis do I have?
- Can you explain my diagnosis as simply as possible?
- How manageable is my type of systemic mastocytosis?
- Is there a cancer center or hospital nearby that specializes in systemic mastocytosis?
- Will I need more testing?

"It's OK to have bad days but don't let yourself stay there. A positive attitude goes a long way."

4

Types of treatment

This chapter presents an overview of the different treatment types for systemic mastocytosis. Together, you and your provider will choose a treatment plan that is best for you.

There are many effective treatments available for systemic mastocytosis. Often this means combinations of medicines that can treat the various symptoms that result from mast cell activation (called anti-mediator drug therapy). Many treatments are listed ahead and in **Guide 2.**

Guide 2 Common treatments for SM (in alphabetical order)
Allogeneic HCT
Antihistamines
Bisphosphonates
Clinical trials
General supportive care
Immunosuppressants
Mast cell stabilizer (cromolyn sodium)
Monoclonal antibody (omalizumab)
Observation
Targeted therapy

Most importantly, treatment starts with talking with your care team who will also help along the way.

Care team

Treatment decisions should involve a multidisciplinary team. This is a team of health care providers from different professional backgrounds who have knowledge (expertise) and experience with systemic mastocytosis. This team is united in the planning and implementation of your treatment. Ask who will coordinate your care.

You know your body better than anyone. Help other team members understand:

- How you feel
- What you need
- What is working and what is not

Once you know who's a part of your care team, you may have many treatment options depending on your symptoms.

Observation

Observation is a plan that closely watches your condition. Observation may also be referred to as surveillance, monitoring, or watch-and-wait. During this time, you will have tests on a regular basis to look for any new or changing symptoms. You will not have any treatment during observation.

Supportive care

Supportive care helps improve your quality of life during and after cancer treatment. The goal is to prevent or manage side effects and symptoms, like pain and cancer-related fatigue. It also addresses the mental, social, and spiritual concerns faced by those with cancer.

Supportive care is available to everyone with cancer and their families, not just those at the end of life. Palliative care is another name for supportive care.

Supportive care can also help with:

- Making treatment decisions
- Coordinating your care
- Paying for care
- Planning for advanced care and end of life

Supportive care can help ease a variety of SM symptoms, including those listed below.

Diarrhea

Diarrhea is frequent and watery bowel movements. Your care team will tell you how to manage diarrhea and may recommend medicines to stop it. It is important to drink lots of fluids. Changes to your diet might help.

Distress

Distress is an unpleasant experience of a mental, physical, social, or spiritual nature. It can affect how you feel, think, and act. Distress might include feelings of sadness, fear, helplessness, worry, anger, and guilt.

Depression, anxiety, and sleeping problems are common in people with cancer. Talk to your provider and with those whom you feel most comfortable about how you are feeling. There are services and people who can help you. Support and counseling services are available.

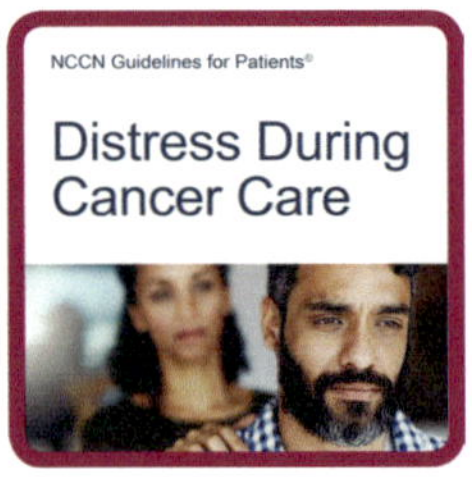

For more information, *see NCCN Guidelines for Patients: Distress During Cancer Care,* available at NCCN.org/patientguidelines and on the NCCN Patient Guides for Cancer app.

Fatigue

Fatigue is a feeling of weariness, tiredness, or a lack of energy. There are treatments for fatigue. Let your care team know how you are feeling and if fatigue is getting in the way of doing the things you enjoy. Eating a balanced diet, exercise, yoga, and massage therapy can help. You might be referred to a dietitian (an expert in nutrition and food) to help with fatigue.

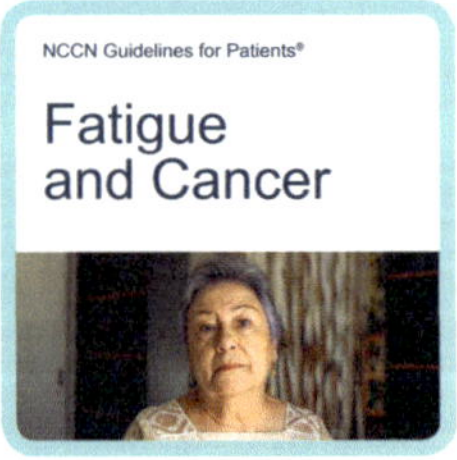

For more information, see *NCCN Guidelines for Patients: Fatigue and Cancer,* available at NCCN.org/patientguidelines and on the NCCN Patient Guides for Cancer app.

Fertility

Fertility is the ability to have children. In order to preserve one's fertility, action may be needed before starting treatment. However, this is not always possible. Those who want to have children in the future should be referred to a fertility specialist to discuss the options.

Nausea and vomiting

Nausea and vomiting could be a sign of systemic mastocytosis. If it happens, you will be given medicine to treat nausea and vomiting. For more information, see *NCCN Guidelines for Patients: Nausea and Vomiting*, available at NCCN.org/patientguidelines and on the NCCN Patient Guides for Cancer app.

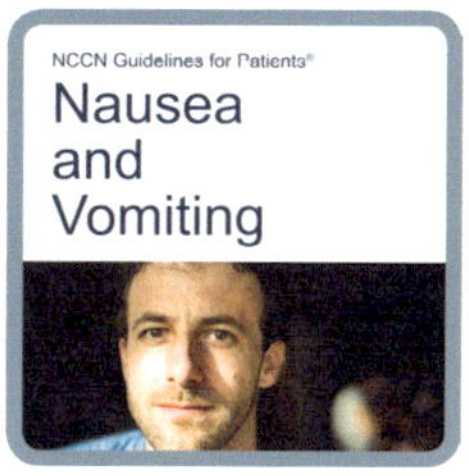

Trouble eating

Sometimes side effects from systemic mastocytosis might cause you to feel not hungry or sick to your stomach (nauseated). You might have a sore mouth. Healthy eating is important during treatment. It includes eating a balanced diet, eating the right amount of food, and drinking enough fluids.

A registered dietitian can help. Speak to your care team if you have trouble eating or maintaining your weight.

Pain

Pain is common in systemic mastocytosis. It might be caused by nausea and vomiting or abdominal cramps from diarrhea. Tell your care team about any pain or discomfort. You might meet with a palliative care specialist or with a pain specialist to manage pain.

Your care team

Treating systemic mastocytosis takes a team of doctors and other experts. Your care team may include:

Dermatologists diagnose and treat skin diseases.

Hematologists diagnose and treat blood diseases and cancers.

Pathologists evaluate and test blood and tissue to diagnose and classify disease.

Gastroenterologists diagnose and treat diseases that occur in the gastrointestinal system.

Allergists diagnose and treat asthma and other allergic diseases.

Immunologists diagnose and treat conditions related to the immune system.

Epinephrine

Epinephrine, also known as adrenaline, is in a class of medicines called alpha- and beta-adrenergic agonists (sympathomimetic agents) used in emergencies to treat allergic reactions. It is a hormone made in the adrenal glands. Epinephrine quickly improves breathing, stimulates the heart, raises dropping blood pressure, reverses hives, and reduces swelling of the face, lips, and throat. One form of epinephrine (EpiPen) you can inject yourself through your skin — often in the thigh — to reverse anaphylaxis (a life-threatening allergic reaction and a medical emergency). NCCN experts recommend always keeping 2 EpiPens with you in case of anaphylaxis.

"Having a chronic, rare disease comes with so much uncertainty. Providers need to be reminded sometimes that the emotional component is real and is as important as the physical one."

Antihistamines

Antihistamines, also referred to as allergy medicine, block histamines to stop allergy symptoms. A histamine is a chemical that your immune system releases to defend against an allergen. Antihistamines are used to treat systemic mastocytosis because many of its symptoms are similar to an allergic reaction. Antihistamines can control itchy skin, watery eyes, as well as other allergic symptoms of SM.

Common antihistamines used for treating symptoms of systemic mastocytosis include:

- Cetirizine hydrochloride (Zyrtec)
- Cimetidine (Tagamet)
- Desloratadine (Clarinex)
- Doxylamine (Unisom)
- Famotidine (Pepcid)
- Fexofenadine (Allegra)
- Hydroxyzine (Atarax, Vistaril)
- Loratadine (Claritin)
- Levocetirizine (Xyzal)

Mast cell stabilizer

Cromolyn sodium is a mast cell stabilizer that helps reduce inflammation. Mast cell stabilizers prevent the release of histamine and other chemical mediators by mast cells. They can be used to prevent or treat a variety of symptoms of systemic mastocytosis. Cromolyn sodium can be taken by mouth, in the form of eye drops, topical ointment, nasal spray, or inhaled with a nebulizer.

Monoclonal antibody

Monoclonal antibody treatment is a type of immunotherapy that can reduce the release of allergy-causing substances in your body. By doing this, it can shrink airway inflammation and make it easier to breathe. Omalizumab (Xolair) is a monoclonal antibody that treats allergic asthma, chronic hives, and food allergies. It is given as an injection by your provider in a hospital or clinic.

Bisphosphonates

Bisphosphonates are medicines that help strengthen bones and prevent bone loss from osteoporosis and other conditions. You might need these if you have a DEXA scan that shows osteoporosis or osteopenia.

Common bisphosphonates include:

- Alendronate (Fosamax)
- Ibandronate (Boniva)
- Risedronate (Actonel)
- Zoledronic acid (Reclast)

Immunosuppressants

Immunosuppressive therapy (IST) uses materials made either by the body or in a lab to improve, target, or restore immune system function. IST is a type of drug therapy that lowers the body's immune response to allow bone marrow stem cells to grow and make new blood cells. Immunosuppressants can be topical (on the skin) or systemic (works throughout your body).

ISTs used to treat systemic mastocytosis include:

- Biologic response modifiers
- Steroids

Biologic response modifiers

Biologic response modifiers (BRMs) are a type of treatment that activates the body's immune system to fight cancer. BRMs are also referred to as immunotherapy. They're used to help the immune system do its job.

Peginterferon alfa-2a (Pegasys), is a specific BRM used to treat systemic mastocytosis. It's an interferon medication that helps regulate

Steroids

In systemic mastocytosis, steroids are used to help reduce allergies and inflammation. The most common types of steroids are tablets, liquid, or intravenous (injection into a vein).

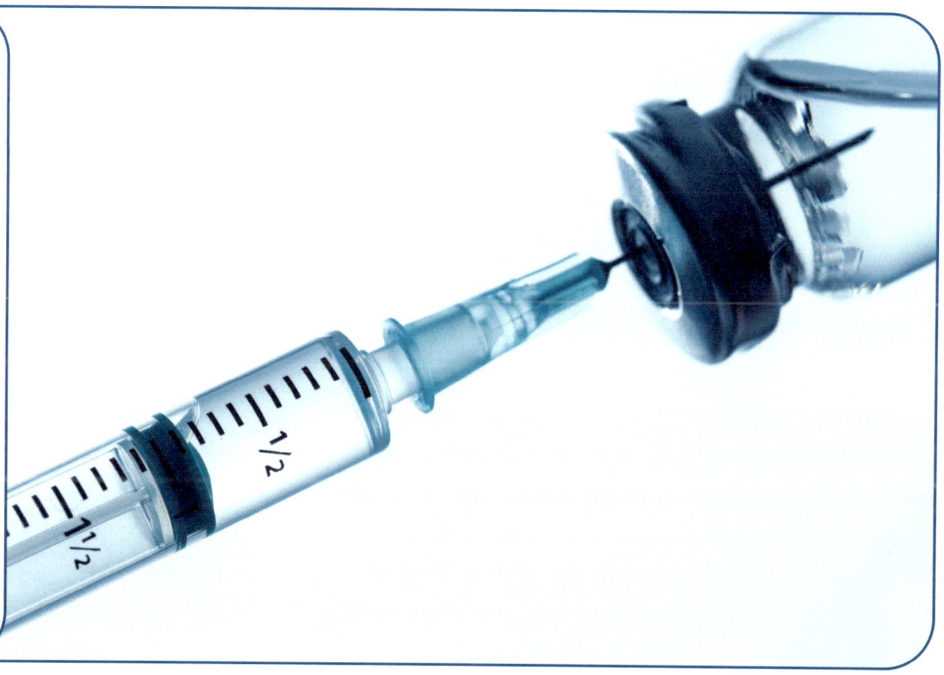

the immune system. Your body makes the protein interferon to help fight viruses. Peginterferon alfa-2a helps boost that ability and can be used in more advanced types of systemic mastocytosis. It's injected into the skin (subcutaneously). It can be used with or without prednisone.

Steroids

Corticosteroids, or steroids, are lab-made immunosuppressants used to reduce inflammation. Steroids can be placed on the skin as an ointment or gel, inhaled through the mouth, used as a mouth (oral) rinse, taken as a pill, or given as an infusion through an IV.

Steroids can cause short-term and long-term side effects. Ask your care team about possible side effects.

Steroids used to treat systemic mastocytosis:

- Prednisone
- Beclomethasone dipropionate (Diprolene)
- Dexamethasone/dexamethasone sodium phosphate
- Hydrocortisone (Cortef)
- Methylprednisolone (Solu-Medrol)

Targeted therapy

Targeted therapy is a form of systemic therapy that works throughout your body. It focuses on specific or unique features of cancer cells. Targeted therapies seek out how cancer cells grow, divide, and move in the body. These drugs stop the action of molecules that help cancer cells grow and/or survive.

Tyrosine kinase inhibitors

A tyrosine kinase inhibitor (TKI) is a type of targeted therapy that blocks the signals that cause cancer to grow and spread. TKIs might be used alone or in combination with other systemic therapies like chemotherapy.

TKIs used to treat systemic mastocytosis include:

- Avapritinib (Ayvakit)
- Imatinib mesylate (Gleevec), if *KIT* mutation negative
- Midostaurin (Rydapt)

Chemotherapy

Chemotherapy kills fast-growing cells throughout the body, including cancer cells and normal cells. Chemotherapy drugs used for the treatment of systemic mastocytosis damage the DNA of cells, which causes them to die.

Cladribine (Leustatin) is a chemotherapy drug used to treat advanced types of systemic mastocytosis. Because of emerging new treatments, leustatin is used less frequently than in the past.

Clinical trials

Another way to receive treatment for SM is through participating in a clinical trial.

A clinical trial is a type of medical research study. After being developed and tested in a lab, potential new ways of fighting cancer need to be studied in people.

If found to be safe and effective in a clinical trial, a drug, device, or treatment approach may be approved by the U.S. Food and Drug Administration (FDA).

Everyone with cancer should carefully consider all of the treatment options available for their cancer type, including standard treatments and clinical trials. Talk to your provider about whether a clinical trial may make sense for you.

Phases

Most cancer clinical trials focus on treatment and are done in phases.

- **Phase 1 trials** study the safety and side effects of an investigational drug or treatment approach.
- **Phase 2 trials** study how well the drug or approach works against a specific type of cancer.
- **Phase 3 trials** test the drug or approach against a standard treatment. If the results are good, it may be approved by the FDA.
- **Phase 4 trials** study the safety and benefit of an FDA-approved treatment.

Who can enroll?

It depends on the clinical trial's rules, called eligibility criteria. The rules may be about age, cancer type and stage, treatment history, or general health. They ensure that participants are alike in specific ways and that the trial is as safe as possible for the participants.

Finding a clinical trial

In the United States

NCCN Cancer Centers
NCCN.org/cancercenters

The National Cancer Institute (NCI)
cancer.gov/about-cancer/treatment/clinical-trials/search

Worldwide

The U.S. National Library of Medicine (NLM)
clinicaltrials.gov/

Need help finding a clinical trial?

NCI's Cancer Information Service (CIS)
1.800.4.CANCER (1.800.422.6237)
cancer.gov/contact

Informed consent

Clinical trials are managed by a research team. This group of experts will review the study with you in detail, including its purpose and the risks and benefits of joining. All of this information is also provided in an informed consent form. Read the form carefully and ask questions before signing it. Take time to discuss it with people you trust. Keep in mind that you can leave and seek treatment outside of the clinical trial at any time.

Will I get a placebo?

Placebos (inactive versions of real medicines) are almost never used alone in cancer clinical trials. It is common to receive either a placebo with a standard treatment or a new drug with a standard treatment. You will be informed, verbally and in writing, if a placebo is part of a clinical trial before you enroll.

Are clinical trials free?

There is no fee to enroll in a clinical trial. The study sponsor pays for research-related costs, including the study drug. But you may need to pay for other services, like transportation or childcare, due to extra appointments. During the trial, you will continue to receive standard cancer care. This care is often covered by insurance.

Allogeneic HCT

Hematopoietic cell transplant (HCT) (also referred to as bone marrow transplant or stem cell transplant) replaces diseased bone marrow with new, healthy blood cells. An allogeneic hematopoietic transplant means it uses healthy stem cells from a donor. The donor may or may not be related to you.

Allogeneic HCT may help cure mast cell diseases, but it is only used in very specific cases because of its risks compared with other effective treatment options.

Before an allogeneic HCT, you will receive a procedure called conditioning. Conditioning uses chemotherapy (and/or radiation therapy) to destroy your bone marrow cells. This procedure creates room for the healthy stem cells and weakens the immune system, so your body does not kill the transplanted cells.

Stem cell transfusion

After conditioning, you will receive the healthy stem cells through a transfusion. This is when blood or parts of blood are slowly pushed through an intravenous (IV) catheter into a vein. This can take several hours.

New, healthy blood cells will form over time. This is called engraftment. It usually occurs about 2 to 4 weeks after the transplant.

Until the new, healthy blood cells form, you will have little or no immune defense. You may need to stay in a very clean room at the hospital or be given antibiotics to prevent or treat infection. While waiting for the cells to engraft, you will likely feel tired and weak.

The procedure carries risks that include infection, bleeding, graft-versus-host disease, secondary cancers, heart complications, and even death.

What's next

This chapter gave an overview of possible treatments for systemic mastocytosis. The next chapter discusses the two most common types: ISM and SSM. They tend to be milder and are treated the same way. For advanced types of systemic mastocytosis, see *Chapter 6: Treatment for SM (advanced).*

Key points

- Treatment decisions should involve a multidisciplinary care team. This is a team of health care providers from different professional backgrounds who have knowledge and experience with systemic mastocytosis.
- Antihistamines, also referred to as allergy medicine, reduce or block histamines to stop allergy symptoms. Antihistamines can control itchy skin, watery eyes, as well as other allergic symptoms of mastocytosis.
- Anaphylaxis is a life-threatening allergic reaction and a medical emergency. NCCN

Allogeneic HCT: Pictured are the steps of a hematopoietic cell transplant.

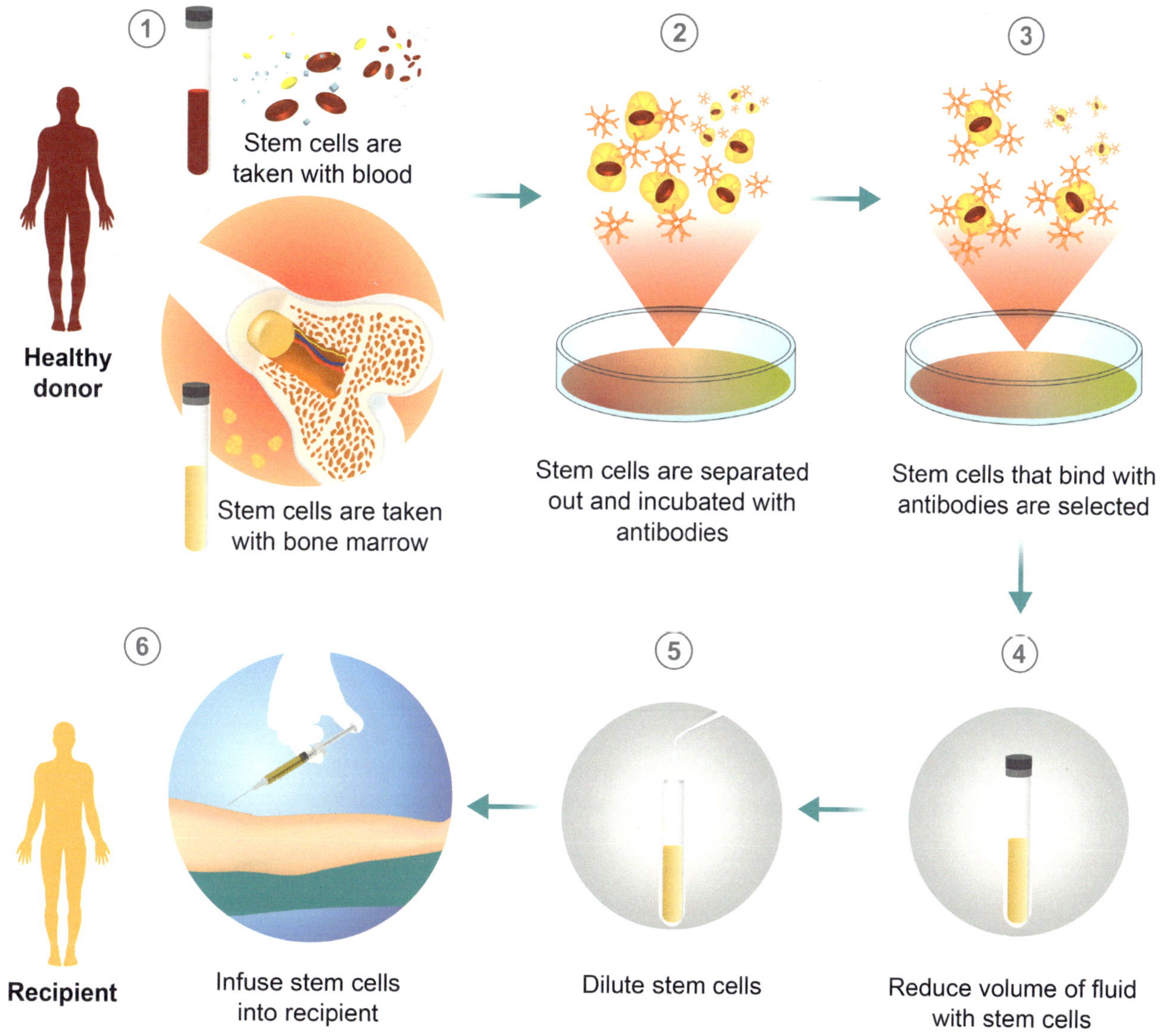

Recipient : (low Immunity system, chemotherapy or radiation therapy)

experts recommend keeping 2 EpiPens with you in case of anaphylaxis.

- Chemotherapy kills fast-growing cells throughout the body, including cancer cells and normal cells.
- Supportive care is health care that relieves symptoms and improves quality of life. It might include pain relief (palliative care), emotional or spiritual support, financial aid, or family counseling.
- Immunosuppressive therapy (IST) uses materials made either by the body or in a laboratory to improve, target, or restore immune system function.
- Observation is a plan that closely watches your condition. You will not have any treatment during observation.

Questions to ask

- What side effects can I expect from treatment?
- Could the treatment affect my fertility or pregnancy? If so, should I speak to a fertility specialist before treatment?
- How often will I need follow-up visits after I finish treatment?
- How will I be involved in making decisions for my treatment?
- Should I bring someone with me to the appointments?

5

Treatment for common types of SM

The more common types of systemic mastocytosis are also milder. They include indolent and smoldering systemic mastocytosis. This chapter focuses on the treatment of those types of SM. You may need ongoing treatment or none at all depending on what's happening with your type of SM.

Indolent systemic mastocytosis (ISM) and smoldering systemic mastocytosis (SMM) are less severe types of SM and are treated the same way. Keep reading to find out how and see **Guide 3.**

ISM and SSM

Indolent systemic mastocytosis

ISM is the most common type of systemic mastocytosis. ISM has a low risk of moving into a more aggressive disease.

ISM refers to an abnormal buildup of mast cells that happens slowly (indolent means chronic without significant worsening). Mast cells build up more often in the bone marrow, as well as other organs or skin. However, the mast cell build up in ISM does not lead to organ problems. Normally functioning organs is what sets ISM apart from more aggressive types of systemic mastocytosis.

ISM can lead to decreased quality of life due to symptoms of mast cell build up and mediator release. Some people with ISM may experience macules (flat and raised) skin lesions (spots), flushing, a swollen liver or spleen, recurrent allergic reactions, or pain and discomfort within the gastrointestinal tract.

Bone marrow mastocytosis (BMM)

BMM is a subtype of ISM and only affects the bone marrow and not the skin or other organs. It is more likely to produce anaphylaxis than ISM. BMM is often linked with osteoporosis, which may be its only symptom.

Guide 3 Possible treatments for ISM and SSM
Referral to centers with expertise in SM
Managing symptoms and triggers
Carry 2 epinephrine self-injectors
Baseline DEXA scan
Skeletal survey
Assess quality of life
Observation
Clinical trial
Avapritinib (for ISM)
Cladribine (useful in some cases)
Peginterferon alfa-2a with or without prednisone (useful in some cases)
Midostaurin (useful in some cases)

Smoldering systemic mastocytosis

SSM is a more severe form of systemic mastocytosis than ISM. SSM refers to a greater buildup of mast cells in your internal organs leading to more symptoms, but this buildup happens slowly (smoldering means moving gradually). People with SSM can remain stable for years, but some can develop a more advanced type of systemic mastocytosis.

Symptoms of SSM typically include swollen lymph nodes, spleen and liver, an increase of mast cells in bone marrow (as seen in anemia or certain cancers), and skin rashes such as urticaria pigmentosa (raised, red, itchy patches).

Treatment options

Because systemic mastocytosis is a rare disorder, your health care provider will likely recommend that you visit a specialized center with providers who have expertise in treating SM. Much of the treatment of ISM and SSM is about managing your symptoms (with what's called anti-mediator drug therapy) and avoiding your specific triggers. Read *Chapter 4: Types of treatment* for the kinds of treatments you might receive as part of anti-mediator drug therapy. To be safe, your provider may encourage you to carry 2 epinephrine self-injectors (EpiPens) to prevent anaphylaxis, which is a severe allergic reaction that can be life threatening.

In addition, you might need a baseline DEXA (dual-x ray absorptiometry) scan to check for signs of osteopenia (weakening bones) or osteoporosis (bone loss). You might also need a metastatic skeletal survey, which is a series of x-rays that check for bone disease throughout your body.

Your provider should also educate you on the signs and symptoms of the disease and assess how they're affecting your quality of life.

Observation

If you remain asymptomatic, which means you're not experiencing any current symptoms, your provider might recommend observation. This is a period of monitoring your health and quality of life and not having any treatment.

During this period, you will have:

- Regular physical examinations
- Blood tests at least annually
- Periodic DEXA scans to check for osteoporosis

Or your provider might suggest you participate in a clinical trial.

Manage triggers and symptoms

If you've been experiencing ISM or SSM symptoms, primary treatment will start with managing them (anti-mediator therapy). For example, you'll be treated using medicines for your specific symptoms like antihistamines, bisphosphonates (bone building drugs), or asthma medicine. Your provider will recommend you always carry 2 epinephrine self-injectors in case of anaphylaxis.

Besides managing triggers and symptoms, the preferred treatment for symptomatic ISM or SSM are the following:

- Clinical trial
- Avapritinib (only for people with ISM who have a normal platelet count)

Preferred therapies have the most evidence they work better and may be safer than other therapies.

Testing after treatment

After the treatment, your care team will want to know how well your treatment is working. So you will see your provider for a physical exam and blood work at least every 6 to 12 months, or sooner if new issues arise.

Your provider will also check the severity of your symptoms and your quality of life. You might also have additional DEXA scans.

If you're responding well to the treatment, then it will be continued.

But if the treatment is not working well or not working at all, then the next preferred treatment is a clinical trial.

Otherwise, you might receive one of the following treatment options that are useful in some cases. Therapies used in certain cases work best for people with specific cancer features or health circumstances. They include:

- Cladribine
- Peginterferon alfa-2a with or without prednisone
- Midostaurin

If testing shows your disease has progressed (worsened), you'll have further testing to find out if your disease is at a more advanced stage. This may include a bone marrow biopsy, bloodwork (serum tryptase testing), and other tests or imaging based on your symptoms. If the tests confirm progression, you'll then be

Even though systemic mastocytosis is a rare disorder, there are many effective treatments available.

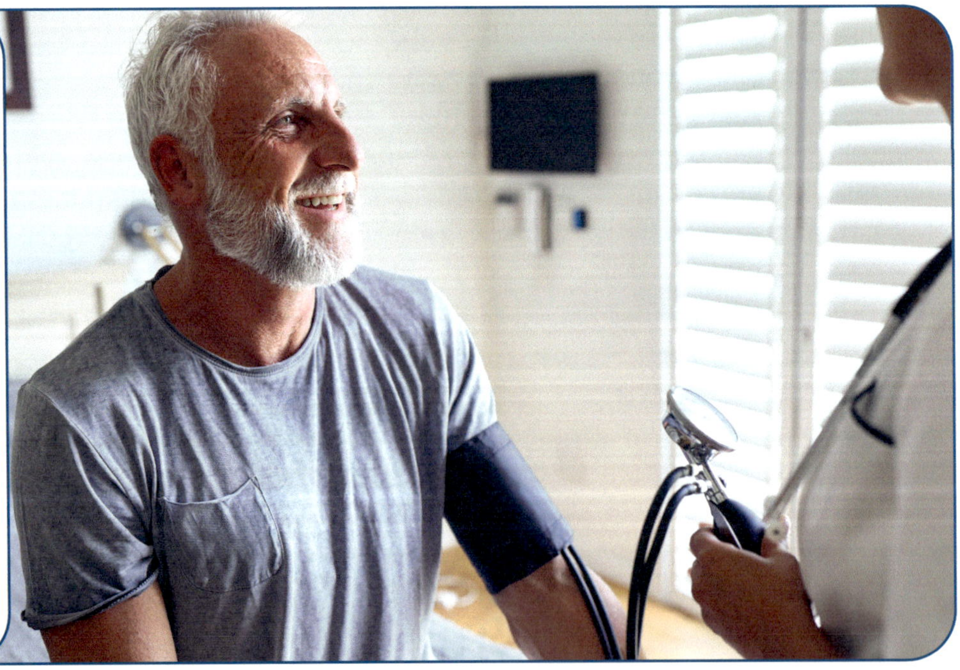

treated based on the new, advanced stage. These include:

- Aggressive systemic mastocytosis
- Systemic mastocytosis with associated hematologic neoplasm (AHN) or SM-AHN
- Mast cell leukemia with or without AHN

More information on advanced types of systemic mastocytosis is in the next chapter.

What's next

This chapter describes the 2 types of systemic mastocytosis that are most common and considered milder: ISM and SSM. The next chapter discusses the 3 advanced types of systemic mastocytosis and how they're treated. These types can form, grow, or spread quicker than the common types and can sometimes be life-threatening.

Key points

- Systemic mastocytosis is often diagnosed by its signs or symptoms.
- Indolent systemic mastocytosis (ISM) is a mild, slow-growing type of systemic mastocytosis.
- Smoldering systemic mastocytosis (SSM) is a type of systemic mastocytosis that has a slow, gradual buildup of mast cells in your internal organs.
- It's important to carry at least 2 EpiPens in case of anaphylaxis.
- If you don't have any symptoms, you will continue with your current treatment.
- If your disease doesn't respond to treatment, it will be restaged to an advanced type of SM.

Questions to ask

- Can I get a copy of the pathology report and other test results?
- Will you explain my pathology report to me?
- Who will talk with me about the next steps? When?
- Should my mast cells be tested for the *KIT* mutation?
- Would you explain my different treatment options and side effects as simply as possible?

"If you don't have access to a specialist in your type of systemic mastocytosis, know that most specialists will do a telehealth consult with your local doctor and you."

6
Treatment for advanced types of SM

Advanced systemic mastocytosis means there is some organ damage. Treatment often involves reducing the number of mast cells in the body. This chapter explains the 3 types of advanced systemic mastocytosis and how they're treated. A clinical trial is a treatment option for any advanced type of SM.

Aggressive systemic mastocytosis

Aggressive systemic mastocytosis (ASM) is when mast cells take over organs and/or bones, resulting in a loss of function (usually liver, gut, bone, or bone marrow). This means you might experience low numbers of white blood cells, anemia, low platelets, liver dysfunction, and bone fractures due to bone lesions.

When systemic mastocytosis is considered aggressive, your provider will likely recommend you go to a center with expertise in treating systemic mastocytosis, if you're not going to one already. Your provider will also make sure you're aware of the signs and the symptoms of the disease and how to avoid its triggers. Also, your care team will suggest you always carry 2 epinephrine self-injectors (EpiPens) in case of anaphylaxis.

Treatment options

Preferred primary treatment options for ASM include:

- Clinical trial
- Avapritinib (for people with a normal platelet count)
- Midostaurin

Other treatment options may include:

- Cladribine
- Peginterferon alfa-2a with or without prednisone
- Imatinib mesylate (used in some cases)

Guide 4 Possible treatments for aggressive systemic mastocytosis
Referral to centers with expertise in SM
Managing symptoms and triggers
Carry 2 epinephrine self-injectors
Clinical trial (preferred)
Avapritinib (preferred for people with 50 or more platelets)
Midostaurin (preferred)
Cladribine (also recommended)
Peginterferon alfa-2a with or without prednisone (also recommended)
Imatinib (for KIT mutation negative, useful in some cases)
Allogeneic HCT

If your mastocytosis responds to primary treatment, your provider may recommend continuing it. Still, depending on any organ damage, your provider might talk to you about having an allogeneic hematopoietic cell transplant (HCT). Because of its risks, allogeneic HCT is only used in some cases.

But if your primary treatment is not working very well or not working at all and you have symptoms of worsening disease, then your disease will be restaged.

Restaging means being retested to find out if your disease is now at a more advanced stage. Tests may include bone marrow biopsy, bloodwork (serum tryptase testing), and other tests or imaging based on your symptoms. If the tests confirm a more advanced stage, then you will be treated based on your new stage of disease.

Your provider might also talk to you about other treatment options that you haven't already tried. Additionally, you and your care team might discuss having an allogeneic HCT.

Systemic mastocytosis with AHN

Systemic mastocytosis with associated hematologic neoplasm (SM-AHN) refers to a mast cell buildup that occurs along with another blood disorder, usually a myelodysplastic syndrome, myeloproliferative disorder, or acute myeloid leukemia (AML). Myeloproliferative neoplasms and myelodysplastic disorders are the most common diseases associated with SM-AHN.

For more information, see *NCCN Guidelines for Patients: Myelodysplastic Syndromes* or *Myeloproliferative Neoplasms*, available at NCCN.org/patientguidelines and on the NCCN Patient Guides for Cancer app.

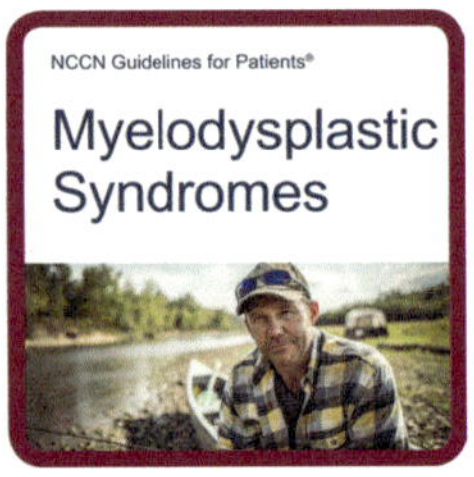

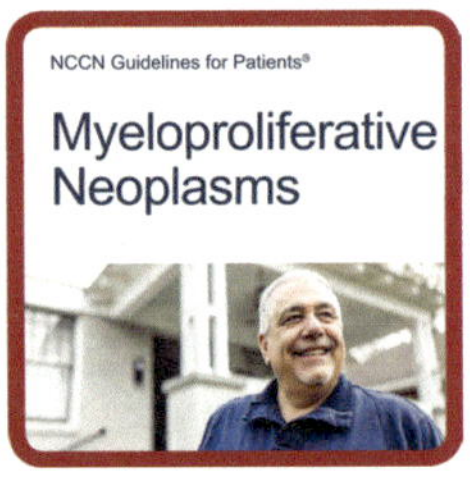

Because a diagnosis of SM-AHN is so rare, your provider may refer you to a specialized center with expertise in mastocytosis, if you're

Guide 5 **Possible treatments for systemic mastocytosis with AHN (SM-AHN)**
Referral to centers with expertise in SM
Managing symptoms and triggers
Carry 2 epinephrine self-injectors
AHN-directed therapy and consideration of allogeneic HCT while managing SM
Clinical trial (preferred)
Avapritinib (preferred, but only if 50 or more platelets)
Midostaurin (preferred)
Cladribine (also recommended)
Peginterferon alfa-2a with or without prednisone
Allogeneic HCT

not going to one already. You'll also be advised to know the signs and symptoms of the disease as well as how to avoid its triggers. And for good measure, your provider will recommend you to always carry 2 epinephrine self-injectors (EpiPens) in case of anaphylaxis.

Treatment options

When you have both SM and AHN, you will work with your care team to decide which condition should be the main focus of treatment.

If AHN is causing more symptoms than SM, then you will have AHN-directed therapy, which includes consideration of an allogeneic HCT. But your SM will also be managed and monitored for any new symptoms or progression of the disease.

However, if SM is causing more symptoms than AHN, the preferred treatments are:

- Clinical trial
- Avapritinib (only for people with a normal platelet count)
- Midostaurin

Other treatment options may include:

- Cladribine
- Peginterferon alfa-2a with or without prednisone

If the treatment reduces your symptoms, your provider may suggest continuing the treatment and/or consider evaluating you for an allogeneic HCT. Because it's a risky procedure, an allogeneic HCT is only used in some cases.

If AHN gets worse, you may be given AHN-directed therapy based on your specific blood disorder. An allogeneic HCT may also be an option while managing the SM.

If your treatment isn't working very well or isn't working at all, and there's evidence of SM-related organ damage or your condition is worse overall, you will undergo more testing to restage your disease. A poor response to treatment means any of the following:

- Return of organ damage or worsening of it
- Swelling of the spleen or liver
- Worsening of systemic mastocytosis symptoms
- Intolerance to drug therapy (too many side effects for you)

Restaging means additional tests, like a bone marrow biopsy, bloodwork (serum tryptase testing), and other tests or imaging, to find out if your disease is now at a more advanced stage. If it is, then you will be treated based on your new stage of disease.

Your provider might consider therapies you haven't already tried and may consider you for an allogeneic HCT if no other treatments seem like a good option.

Mast cell leukemia with or without AHN

Mast cell leukemia (MCL) is the rarest and most aggressive (fast-growing) type of systemic mastocytosis. MCL leads to the buildup of immature mast cells in more than one-fifth of your body's tissues or organs. This buildup of abnormal mast cells can cause severe organ damage and bone pain. Although MCL has a poor prognosis (outlook) and it can be life-threatening, the prognosis is improving with many treatments being available.

What is leukemia?

Leukemia is a cancer caused by cells in your bone marrow that overproduce abnormal or underdeveloped blood cells. There are many types of leukemia, each based on the type of blood cells that are affected.

MCL is a rare type of leukemia identified by an abnormal growth of immature mast cells in the bone marrow.

MCL with AHN

MCL with associated hematologic neoplasm (AHN) is a leukemia diagnosis that includes another blood disorder, usually myelodysplastic syndrome, myeloproliferative neoplasms (myeloproliferative disorders), or AML. The prognosis tends to be worse in people who have MCL with AHN than just MCL.

There is no clear reason why MCL develops, but several mutations in the *KIT* gene have been linked to it. It can arise suddenly (called de novo) or as a progression of systemic mastocytosis.

Symptoms of MCL may include:

- Hot flashes
- Fever
- Rapid heartbeat
- Low blood pressure
- Losing more than one-tenth body weight
- Fatigue

Symptoms related to organ involvement:

- Bone pain or fractures
- Diarrhea and other gastrointestinal issues

Guide 6 Possible treatments for mast cell leukemia with or without AHN
Referral to centers with expertise in SM
Managing symptoms and triggers
Carry 2 epinephrine self-injectors
Clinical trial (preferred)
Avapritinib (preferred, but only if 50 or more platelets)
Midostaurin (preferred)
Cladribine (also recommended)
AML-based therapy with consideration of cladribine or midostaurin
Allogeneic HCT
AHN-directed therapy

If you have a diagnosis of MCL with or without AHN, your care team may refer you to specialized centers with expertise in mastocytosis, if you're not going to one already. They'll recommend you know the signs and symptoms of the disease as well as its triggers. Your care team will also advise you to always carry 2 epinephrine self-injectors (EpiPens) in case of anaphylaxis.

Treatment options

Preferred treatment options for MCL include:

- Clinical trial
- Avapritinib
- Midostaurin

Other treatment options may include:

- Cladribine
- Acute myeloid leukemia-based therapy with consideration of cladribine or midostaurin

If your primary treatment is effective, you may be asked to continue it and/or consider an allogeneic HCT.

If your disease gets worse (progresses to AHN or transforms into acute myeloid leukemia), you may be given AHN-directed therapy. AHN-directed therapy is based on your specific hematologic neoplasm and may have more specific treatments. It may include multiagent chemotherapy (a combination of chemotherapy drugs) and/or consideration of an allogeneic HCT while managing MCL.

For more information, see *NCCN Guidelines for Patients: Acute Myeloid Leukemia,* available at NCCN.org/patientguidelines and on the NCCN Patient Guides for Cancer app.

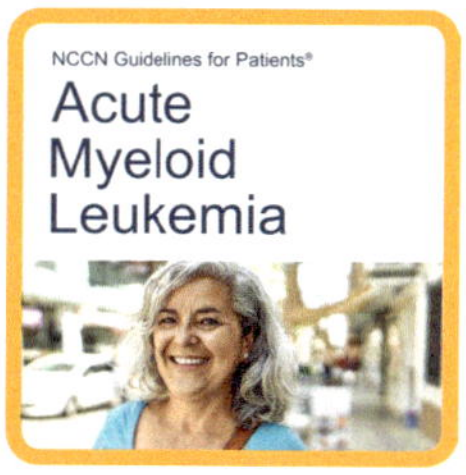

If your treatment is not working very well or not working at all, you can undergo more testing to restage your disease. When your disease is restaged, your provider might suggest a treatment you haven't tried before and/or an allogeneic HCT.

Any of the following can happen if treatment isn't working:

- Return of organ damage or worsening of it
- Swelling of the spleen or liver
- Worsening of systemic mastocytosis symptoms
- Intolerance to drug therapy (too many side effects for you)

Treatment at this stage will often focus on supportive care. This includes symptom relief, an emphasis on quality of life, and longer survival. It is important to ask your health care provider about your prognosis. See *Chapter 4: Types of treatment* for more information on how supportive care can help.

If you're feeling stress or anxiety related to your cancer, you're not alone and help is available. For more information about coping with distress related to your cancer, read *NCCN Guidelines for Patients: Distress During Cancer Care* at NCCN.org/patientguidelines and on the NCCN Patient Guides for Cancer app.

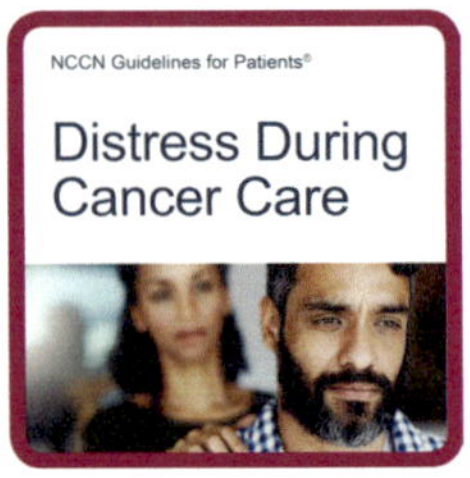

What's next

This chapter details the advanced forms of systemic mastocytosis and their treatment. A chronic, progressive disease like advanced systemic mastocytosis can be difficult to deal with due to the many unknowns. You may want more information so be sure to read the next chapter that provides ideas on helpful resources.

Key points

- Aggressive systemic mastocytosis is described as a loss of organ function (usually liver, gut, bone, or bone marrow) due to mast cells taking over.
- When you have both SM and an associated hematologic neoplasm, you will work with your care team to decide which condition should be the main focus of treatment.
- Participating in a clinical trial is always an option for people with advanced SM.
- For any advanced type of SM, an allogeneic HCT may be considered after trying other treatments.
- Mast cell leukemia (MCL) is a very rare and aggressive type of systemic mastocytosis.
- There is no clear reason why MCL develops, but several mutations in the *KIT* gene have been linked to it.

Questions to ask

- Will my age, health, and other factors affect my treatment options?
- What is the goal of each treatment?
- What support is available to me?
- Can I stop treatment at any time?
- What will happen if I stop treatment?

7 Other resources

Want to learn more? Here's how you can get additional help.

What else to know

This book can help you improve your cancer care. It plainly explains expert recommendations and suggests questions to ask your care team. But it's not the only resource that you have.

You're welcome to receive as much information and help as you need. Many people are interested in learning more about:

- The details of their systemic mastocytosis and treatment
- Being a part of a care team
- Getting financial help
- Finding a care provider who is an expert in systemic mastocytosis
- Coping with health problems

What else to do

Your health care center can help you with next steps. They often have on-site resources to help meet your needs and find answers to your questions. Health care centers can also inform you of resources in your community.

In addition to help from your providers, the resources listed in the next section provide support for many people like yourself. Look through the list and visit the provided websites to learn more about these organizations.

Where to get help

CancerCare
Cancercare.org

Imerman Angels
Imermanangels.org

National Coalition for Cancer Survivorship
Canceradvocacy.org

TargetCancer Foundation
Targetcancer.org

The Leukemia & Lymphoma Society
LLS.org/PatientSupport

The Mast Cell Disease Society
tmsforacure.org

Triage Cancer
triagecancer.org

Questions to ask

- Who can I talk to about help with housing, food, and other basic needs?
- What assistance is available for transportation, childcare, and home care?
- How much will I have to pay for treatment?
- What help is available to pay for medicines and other treatment?
- What other services are available to me and my caregivers (like translation services)?

"Never. Lose. Hope. Tomorrow could be the day you have been waiting for."

We want your feedback!

Our goal is to provide helpful and easy-to-understand information on cancer. Take our survey to let us know what we got right and what we could do better. NCCN.org/patients/feedback

Words to know

acute myeloid leukemia (AML)
A fast-growing cancer that starts in the bone marrow and causes too many young white blood cells to be made.

allogeneic hematopoietic cell transplant
A cancer treatment that replaces abnormal blood stem cells with healthy donor cells.

anemia
A health condition in which the amount of healthy red blood cells is too low to carry enough oxygen to the rest of your body.

anti-mediator therapy
Treatments that help lessen the release (and the effects) of mast cell mediators, like histamine.

antihistamines
A medicine that reduces or blocks histamines to stop allergy symptoms. It can control itchy skin, watery eyes, as well as other allergic symptoms of mastocytosis.

biopsy
Removal of small amounts of tissue from your body to test for disease.

blood stem cell
A blood-forming cell from which all other types of blood cells are formed. Also called a hematopoietic stem cell.

bone marrow
The sponge-like tissue in the center of most bones where blood cells are formed.

bone marrow aspiration
The removal of a small amount of liquid bone marrow to test for disease.

chemotherapy
Drugs that kill fast-growing cells, including normal cells and cancer cells.

clinical trial
A research study of how safe and helpful new tests and treatments are for people with a specific condition.

complete blood count (CBC)
A lab test that measures the number of blood cells.

contrast
A substance put into your body to make clearer pictures during imaging tests.

cytogenetic testing
A test that uses a microscope to examine a cell's chromosomes.

dermatologist
A doctor who specializes in the diagnosis and treatment of skin diseases.

DNA
A chain of chemicals in cells that contain coded instructions for making and controlling cells.

diagnosis
Identification of a disease based on tests.

differential
A measure of the different types of white blood cells present in a blood sample.

fatigue
Severe tiredness that limits the ability to function.

fluorescence in situ hybridization (FISH)
A lab test that uses special dyes to look for abnormal changes in a cell's genes and chromosomes.

gene
A set of coded instructions in cells for making and controlling cells.

hematopoietic cell transplant (HCT)
A type of treatment that destroys cells in the bone marrow, then replaces them with new, healthy blood-forming cells. Also called stem cell transplant or bone marrow transplant.

human leukocyte antigen (HLA)
A cell protein that helps your body know its own cells from foreign cells.

immune system
The body's natural defense against infection and disease.

immunotherapy
A medicine that increases the activity of your body's disease-fighting system.

liver function tests
Tests that measure chemicals made or processed by the liver.

mast cell
A cell of the immune system responsible for allergic reactions and immune responses.

mast cell activation
When mast cells release a large amount of mediators, like histamine.

mast cell mediators
Molecules that are released when mast cells activate. They're responsible for inflammation and allergic reactions. Histamine and tryptase are mast cell mediators.

myelodysplastic syndromes (MDS)
A group of rare bone marrow disorders.

myeloproliferative neoplasm (MPN)
A cancer in which the bone marrow makes too many red blood cells, white blood cells, or platelets.

mutation
A change in a gene that alters the genetic message carried by that gene.

palliative care
Specialized medical care aimed at increasing quality of life and reducing pain and discomfort for people with serious, complex illness.

pathologist
A doctor who is an expert in testing cells and tissue to find disease.

platelet
A type of blood cell that helps control bleeding. Also called a thrombocyte.

red blood cell
A type of blood cell that carries oxygen from the lungs to the rest of the body. Also called an erythrocyte.

side effect
An unhealthy or unpleasant physical or emotional response to treatment.

supportive care
Care that includes symptom relief but not cancer treatment. Also called palliative care.

systemic therapy
Treatment that works throughout the body.

targeted therapy
A drug treatment that identifies and attacks a specific feature of cancer cells with less harm to normal cells.

white blood cell
A type of blood cell that helps fight infections in the body. Also called a leukocyte.

NCCN Contributors

This patient guide is based on the NCCN Clinical Practice Guidelines in Oncology (NCCN Guidelines®) for Systemic Mastocytosis, Version 1.2025. It was adapted, reviewed, and published with help from the following people:

Dorothy A. Shead, MS
Senior Director
Patient Information Operations

Christine McLaughlin
Medical Writer

Susan Kidney
Senior Graphic Design Specialist

The NCCN Clinical Practice Guidelines in Oncology (NCCN Guidelines®) for Systemic Mastocytosis, Version 1.2025 were developed by the following NCCN Panel Members:

Aaron T. Gerds, MD, MS/Chair
Case Comprehensive Cancer Center/ UniversityHospitals Seidman Cancer Center and Cleveland Clinic Taussig Cancer Institute

Jason Gotlib, MD, MS/Vice-Chair
Stanford Cancer Institute

Peter Abdelmessieh, DO, MSc
Fox Chase Cancer Center

Haris Ali, MD
City of Hope National Medical Center

Mariana Castells, MD, PhD
Adjunct Panel Member
Dana-Farber/Brigham and Women's Cancer Center

*Ruth Fein Revell, BS
Patient Advocate

Steven Green, MD
Roswell Park Comprehensive Cancer Center

Krishna Gundabolu, MBBS, MS
Fred & Pamela Buffett Cancer Center

Elizabeth Hexner, MD, MS
Abramson Cancer Center at the University of Pennsylvania

Tania Jain, MBBS
Johns Hopkins Kimmel Cancer Center

Catriona H. Jamieson, MD, PhD
UC San Diego Moores Cancer Center

Paul R. Kaesberg, MD
UC Davis Comprehensive Cancer Center

Irum Khan, MD
Robert H. Lurie Comprehensive Cancer Center of Northwestern University

*Andrew T. Kuykendall, MD
Moffitt Cancer Center

Yazan F. Madanat, MD
UT Southwestern Simmons Comprehensive Cancer Center

Naveen Manchanda, MD
Indiana University Melvin and Bren Simon Comprehensive Cancer Center

Lucia Masarova, MD
The University of Texas MD Anderson Cancer Center

Jori May, MD
O'Neal Comprehensive Cancer Center at UAB

Brandon McMahon, MD
University of Colorado Cancer Center

Sanjay R. Mohan, MD, MSCI
Vanderbilt-Ingram Cancer Center

Kalyan V. Nadiminti, MD
University of Wisconsin Carbone Cancer Center

Stephen Oh, MD, PhD
Siteman Cancer Center at Barnes-Jewish Hospital and Washington University School of Medicine

Jeanne Palmer, MD
Mayo Clinic Comprehensive Cancer Center

Ami B. Patel, MD
Huntsman Cancer Institute at the University of Utah

Anand A. Patel, MD
The UChicago Medicine Comprehensive Cancer Center

Nikolai Podoltsev, MD, PhD
Yale Cancer Center/Smilow Cancer Hospital

*Lindsay Rein, MD
Duke Cancer Institute

Rachel Salit, MD
Fred Hutchinson Cancer Center

Mary Sehl, MD
UCLA Jonsson Comprehensive Cancer Center

Moshe Talpaz, MD
University of Michigan Rogel Cancer Center

*Martha Wadleigh, MD
Dana-Farber/Brigham and Women's Cancer Center

Sarah A. Wall, MD, MPH
The Ohio State University Comprehensive Cancer Center - James Cancer Hospital and Solove Research Institute

NCCN

Mary Anne Bergman
Guidelines Coordinator

Cindy Hochstetler, PhD
Oncology Scientist/Senior Medical Writer

* Reviewed this patient guide. For disclosures, visit NCCN.org/disclosures.

NCCN Cancer Centers

Abramson Cancer Center
at the University of Pennsylvania
Philadelphia, Pennsylvania
800.789.7366 • *pennmedicine.org/cancer*

Case Comprehensive Cancer Center/
University Hospitals Seidman Cancer Center and
Cleveland Clinic Taussig Cancer Institute
Cleveland, Ohio
UH Seidman Cancer Center
800.641.2422 • *uhhospitals.org/services/cancer-services*
CC Taussig Cancer Institute
866.223.8100 • *my.clevelandclinic.org/departments/cancer*
Case CCC
216.844.8797 • *case.edu/cancer*

City of Hope National Medical Center
Duarte, California
800.826.4673 • *cityofhope.org*

Dana-Farber/Brigham and Women's Cancer Center |
Mass General Cancer Center
Boston, Massachusetts
877.442.3324 • *youhaveus.org*
617.726.5130 • *massgeneral.org/cancer-center*

Duke Cancer Institute
Durham, North Carolina
888.275.3853 • *dukecancerinstitute.org*

Fox Chase Cancer Center
Philadelphia, Pennsylvania
888.369.2427 • *foxchase.org*

Fred & Pamela Buffett Cancer Center
Omaha, Nebraska
402.559.5600 • *unmc.edu/cancercenter*

Fred Hutchinson Cancer Center
Seattle, Washington
206.667.5000 • *fredhutch.org*

Huntsman Cancer Institute at the University of Utah
Salt Lake City, Utah
800.824.2073 • *healthcare.utah.edu/huntsmancancerinstitute*

Indiana University Melvin and Bren Simon
Comprehensive Cancer Center
Indianapolis, Indiana
888.600.4822 • *www.cancer.iu.edu*

Johns Hopkins Kimmel Cancer Center
Baltimore, Maryland
410.955.8964
www.hopkinskimmelcancercenter.org

Mayo Clinic Comprehensive Cancer Center
Phoenix/Scottsdale, Arizona
Jacksonville, Florida
Rochester, Minnesota
480.301.8000 • Arizona
904.953.0853 • Florida
507.538.3270 • Minnesota
mayoclinic.org/cancercenter

Memorial Sloan Kettering Cancer Center
New York, New York
800.525.2225 • *mskcc.org*

Moffitt Cancer Center
Tampa, Florida
888.663.3488 • *moffitt.org*

O'Neal Comprehensive Cancer Center at UAB
Birmingham, Alabama
800.822.0933 • *uab.edu/onealcancercenter*

Robert H. Lurie Comprehensive Cancer Center
of Northwestern University
Chicago, Illinois
866.587.4322 • *cancer.northwestern.edu*

Roswell Park Comprehensive Cancer Center
Buffalo, New York
877.275.7724 • *roswellpark.org*

Siteman Cancer Center at Barnes-Jewish Hospital
and Washington University School of Medicine
St. Louis, Missouri
800.600.3606 • *siteman.wustl.edu*

St. Jude Children's Research Hospital/
The University of Tennessee Health Science Center
Memphis, Tennessee
866.278.5833 • *stjude.org*
901.448.5500 • *uthsc.edu*

Stanford Cancer Institute
Stanford, California
877.668.7535 • *cancer.stanford.edu*

The Ohio State University Comprehensive Cancer Center -
James Cancer Hospital and Solove Research Institute
Columbus, Ohio
800.293.5066 • *cancer.osu.edu*

The UChicago Medicine Comprehensive Cancer Center
Chicago, Illinois
773.702.1000 • *uchicagomedicine.org/cancer*

The University of Texas MD Anderson Cancer Center
Houston, Texas
844.269.5922 • *mdanderson.org*

UC Davis Comprehensive Cancer Center
Sacramento, California
916.734.5959 • 800.770.9261
health.ucdavis.edu/cancer

UC San Diego Moores Cancer Center
La Jolla, California
858.822.6100 • cancer.ucsd.edu

UCLA Jonsson Comprehensive Cancer Center
Los Angeles, California
310.825.5268 • uclahealth.org/cancer

UCSF Helen Diller Family
Comprehensive Cancer Center
San Francisco, California
800.689.8273 • cancer.ucsf.edu

University of Colorado Cancer Center
Aurora, Colorado
720.848.0300 • coloradocancercenter.org

University of Michigan Rogel Cancer Center
Ann Arbor, Michigan
800.865.1125 • rogelcancercenter.org

University of Wisconsin Carbone Cancer Center
Madison, Wisconsin
608.265.1700 • uwhealth.org/cancer

UT Southwestern Simmons
Comprehensive Cancer Center
Dallas, Texas
214.648.3111 • utsouthwestern.edu/simmons

Vanderbilt-Ingram Cancer Center
Nashville, Tennessee
877.936.8422 • vicc.org

Yale Cancer Center/Smilow Cancer Hospital
New Haven, Connecticut
855.4.SMILOW • yalecancercenter.org

share with us.

Take our survey and help make the NCCN Guidelines for Patients better for everyone!

NCCN.org/patients/comments

Index

Made in the USA
Middletown, DE
16 September 2026

33225902R00033